MEASLES CURE

A step to step guide on things you need to know to treat measles

Dr Rowan Theo

Table of Contents

CHAPTER ONE

measles
Everything You Need to Know About the Measles

Measles, or rubella, is a viral contamination that begins offevolved in the respiration gadget. It nonetheless stays a substantial purpose of dying worldwide, notwithstanding the supply of a safe, powerful vaccine.

Measles signs

Symptoms of measles usually first seem inside 10 to twelve days of publicity to the virus. They consist of:

- cough

- fever

- runny nostril

- pink eyes

- sore throat

- white spots in the mouth

A big pores and skin rash is a conventional signal of measles. This rash can last as long as 7 days and usually seems inside 14 days of publicity to the virus. It generally develops on the top and slowly spreads to different elements of the frame.

Measles reasons

Measles is because of contamination with an endemic from the paramyxovirus family. Viruses are tiny parasitic microbes. Once you've been inflamed, the virus invades host cells and makes use of mobile additives to finish its existence cycle.

The measles virus infects the respiration tract first. However, it finally spreads to different elements of the frame via the bloodstream.

Measles is most effective acknowledged to arise in people and now no longer in different animals. There are 24known genetic styles of measles, despite the fact that most effective 6 are presently circulating.

Is measles airborne?

Measles may be unfold via the air from respiration droplets and small aerosol debris. An inflamed man or woman can launch the virus into the air after they cough or sneeze.

These respiration debris also can determine items and surfaces. You can come to be inflamed in case you come into touch with a infected object, along with a door handle, after which contact your face, nostril, or mouth.

The measles virus can stay outdoor of the frame for longer than you could think. In fact, it is able to continue to be infectious in the air or on surfaces for up to 2 hours.

Is measles contagious?

Measles is enormously contagious. This way that the contamination can unfold very without problems from man or woman to man or woman.

A prone man or woman that's uncovered to the measles virus has a ninety percentage hazard of turning into inflamed. Additionally, an inflamed man or woman can move directly to unfold the virus to everywhere among nine and 18susceptible people.

A man or woman that has measles can unfold the virus to others earlier than they even understand that they have got it. An inflamed man or woman is contagious for 4 days earlier than the function rash seems. After the rash seems, they're nonetheless contagious for every other 4 days.

The primary chance element for catching measles is being

unvaccinated. Additionally, a few corporations are at a better chance of growing headaches from measles contamination, together with younger youngsters, humans with a weakened immune gadget, and pregnant ladies.

Diagnosing measles

If you observed which you have measles or were uncovered to a person with measles, touch your physician immediately. They can examine you and direct you wherein to be visible to decide when you have the contamination.

Doctors can affirm measles with the aid of using analyzing your pores and skin rash and checking for signs which are function of the disorder, along with white spots in the mouth, fever, cough, and sore throat.

If they think you could have measles primarily based totally to your records and observation, your physician will order a blood take a look at to test for the measles virus.

CHAPTER TWO

Treatment for measles

There's no particular remedy for measles. Unlike bacterial infections, viral infections aren't touchy to antibiotics. The virus and signs commonly disappear in approximately or 3 weeks.

There are a few interventions to be had for individuals who may also were uncovered to the virus. These can assist save you an contamination or reduce its severity. They consist of:

• a measles vaccine, given inside seventy two hours of publicity

- a dose of immune proteins referred to as immunoglobulin, taken inside six days of publicity

Your physician may also suggest the subsequent that will help you get better:

- acetaminophen (Tylenol) or ibuprofen (Advil) to lessen fever

- relaxation to assist enhance your immune gadget

- masses of fluids

- a humidifier to ease a cough and sore throat

- diet A supplements

Measles in babies

The measles vaccine isn't given to youngsters till they're at the least three hundred and sixty five days old. Before receiving their first dose of the vaccine is the time they're maximum susceptible to being inflamed with the measles virus.

Babies acquire a few safety from measles via passive immunity, that's furnished from mom to infant via the placenta and throughout breastfeeding.

However, studies has proven that this immunity may be misplaced in only over 2.five months after start or the time breastfeeding is discontinued.

Children under five years of age are much more likely to have headaches because of measles. These can consist of such things as pneumonia, encephalitis, and ear infections that may bring about listening to loss.

Incubation duration for measles

The incubation duration of an infectious disorder is the time that passes among publicity and whilst signs expand. The incubation duration for measles is among 10 and 14 days.

After the preliminary incubation duration, you could start to revel in nonspecific signs, along with fever, cough, and runny nostril. The rash will start to expand numerous days later.

It's crucial to don't forget that you could nonetheless unfold the contamination to others for 4 days previous to growing the rash. If you suspect you've been uncovered to measles and haven't been vaccinated, you have to touch your physician as quickly as possible.

Measles types

In addition to a conventional measles contamination, there also are numerous different styles of measles infections that you could get.

Atypical measles takes place in individuals who acquired a killed measles vaccine. When uncovered to measles, those people come down with an contamination that has signs along with excessive fever, rash, and on occasion pneumonia.

Modified measles takes place in individuals who've been given post-publicity immunoglobulin and in toddlers who nonetheless have a few passive immunity. Modified measles is commonly milder than a ordinary case of measles.

Hemorrhagic measles is hardly ever pronounced in the United States. It reasons signs like excessive fever, seizures, and bleeding into the pores and skin and mucus membranes.

CHAPTER THREE

Measles vs. rubella

You may also have heard rubella stated as "German measles." But measles and rubella are simply because of distinctive viruses.

Rubella isn't as contagious as measles. However, it is able to purpose severe headaches if a lady develops the contamination at the same time as pregnant.

Even aleven though distinctive viruses purpose measles and rubella, they're additionally comparable in numerous approaches. Both viruses:

- may be unfold via the air from coughing and sneezing

- purpose fever and a exclusive rash

- arise most effective in people

Both measles and rubella are covered in the measles-mumps-rubella (MMR) and measles-mumps-rubella-varicella (MMRV) vaccines.

Measles prevention

There some approaches to save you turning into unwell with measles.

Vaccination

Getting vaccinated is the nice manner to save you measles. Two doses of the measles vaccine are ninety seven percentage powerful at stopping measles contamination.

There are vaccines to be had — the MMR vaccine and the MMRV vaccine. The MMR vaccine is a 3-in-one vaccination that may guard you from measles, mumps, and rubella. The MMRV vaccine protects in opposition to the identical infections because the MMR vaccine and additionally consists of safety in opposition to chickenpox.

Children can acquire their first vaccination at three hundred and sixty five days, or quicker if travelling internationally, and their 2nd dose among the a while of four and 6. Adults who've in no way acquired an immunization can request the vaccine from their physician.

Some corporations shouldn't acquire a vaccination in opposition to measles. These corporations consist of:

• individuals who've had a preceding existencc-threatening response to the measles vaccine or its additives

• pregnant ladies

• immunocompromised people, that may consist of humans with HIV or AIDS, humans present process most cancers remedy, or humans on medicines that suppress the immune gadget

Side results to vaccination are commonly moderate and disappear in some days. They can consist of such things as fever and moderate rash. In uncommon cases, the vaccine has been related to low platelet depend or seizures. Most youngsters and adults who acquire a measles vaccine don't revel in aspect results.

Some accept as true with that the measles vaccine can purpose autism in youngsters. As a result, an extreme quantity of look at has been dedicated to this subject matter over many years. This studies has located that there may be no link between vaccines and autism.

Vaccination isn't simply crucial for defensive you and your family. It's additionally crucial for defensive individuals who can't be vaccinated. When extra humans are vaccinated in opposition to a disorder, it's much less in all likelihood to flow into in the populace. This is referred to as herd immunity.

To reap herd immunity in opposition to measles, about ninety six percentage of the populace ought to be vaccinated.

Other prevention methods

Not anyone can acquire the measles vaccination. But there are different approaches that you could assist to save you the unfold of measles.

If you're prone to contamination:

• Practice correct hand hygiene. Wash your fingers earlier than consuming, after the usage of the bathroom, and earlier than touching your face, mouth, or nostril.

• Don't percentage private gadgets with individuals who can be unwell. This can consist of such things as consuming utensils, consuming glasses, and toothbrushes.

• Avoid entering touch with individuals who are unwell

If you're unwell with measles:

• Stay domestic from paintings or faculty and different public locations till you aren't contagious.

This is 4 days once you first expand the measles rash.

• Avoid touch with individuals who can be susceptible to contamination, along with toddlers too younger to be vaccinated and immunocompromised humans.

• Cover your nostril and mouth in case you want to cough or sneeze. Dispose of all used tissues promptly. If you don't have a tissue to be had, sneeze into the criminal of your elbow, now no longer into your hand.

• Be certain to scrub your fingers
often and to disinfect any surfaces
or items which you contact often.

CHAPTER FOUR

Measles throughout being pregnant

Pregnant ladies who don't have immunity to measles have to take care to keep away from publicity throughout their being pregnant. Coming down with measles throughout your being pregnant may have substantial terrible fitness results on each the mom and fetus.

Pregnant ladies are at an multiplied chance for headaches from measles along with pneumonia. Additionally, having measles at the same time as pregnant can cause the subsequent being pregnant headaches:

• miscarriage

• preterm labor

• low start weight

• stillbirth

Measles also can be transmitted from mom to infant if the mom has measles near her transport date. This is referred to as congenital measles. Babies with congenital measles have a rash after start or expand one quickly afterward. They're at an multiplied chance of headaches, which may be existence-threatening.

If you're pregnant, don't have immunity to measles, and accept as true with which you've been uncovered, you have to touch your physician immediately. Receiving an injection of immunoglobulin may also assist to save you an contamination.

Measles prognosis

Measles has a low dying fee in healthful youngsters and adults, and maximum individuals who agreement the measles virus get better fully. The chance of headaches is better in the following corporations:

• youngsters under five years old

• adults over twenty years old

• pregnant ladies

• humans with a weakened immune gadget

• those who are malnourished

• humans with a diet A deficiency

Approximately 30 percentage of humans with measles revel in one or extra headaches. Measles can cause existence-threatening headaches, along with pneumonia and infection of the brain (encephalitis).

Other headaches related to measles may also consist of:

• ear contamination

- bronchitis

- croup

- excessive diarrhea

- blindness

- being pregnant headaches, along with miscarriage or preterm labor

- subacute sclerosing panencephalitis (SSPE), an extraordinary degenerative situation of the fearful gadget that develops years after contamination

It is enormously not going which you get measles extra than once. After you've got had the virus, your frame has advanced immunity in opposition to the contamination.

However, measles and its capacity headaches are preventable via vaccination. Vaccination now no longer most effective protects you and your family, however additionally prevents the measles virus from circulating to your network and affecting folks who can't be vaccinated.

THE END